ULTIMATE SUPERFOODS VOL.1

– THE INDIAN GOOSEBERRY:

HOW TO BOOST YOUR BODY'S IMMUNE SYSTEM BY INGESTING AMLA, AMALAKI, TRIPHALA, AND CHYAVANPRASH

DR. CALVIN CLIDE, Ph.D

DEDICATION

I, Dr. Calvin Clide, Ph.D hereby dedicate this book and all its contents to everyone in the world and hope that it can be a great revelation to those who are seeking new ways to better their health and create longevity in their lives. I'd like to thank the ones who supported me along my journey in life and would like to thank my colleague and business partner, Maxwell Louis, specifically, for giving me the idea to write out this series. What you are witnessing is years of accumulation of knowledge from the world's most powerful superfoods, which I have been using to help my grandmother, a woman of many ailments, and my loved ones heal during times of need, now, I am sharing it with you, the world, and all its inhabitants. May we all be blessed with the Sacred Knowledge of Life, Health, and Longevity! This is Ultimate Superfoods VOL. 1, the first of many volumes to come. I really hope you enjoy reading this as much as I enjoyed writing it. I put a lot of time and energy into this series and I hope that it can be transmuted to divine inspiration and wisdom for those seeking new avenues of life. Thank you, Dear reader, for you mean the world to me!

CONTENTS

ACKNOWLEDGMENTS

I want to take this time to acknowledge my mother, who is the reason I strive so hard to better myself and the world around me, she is my light, she is my joy, and I will always keep her in my heart.

INTRODUCTION

In this book you will find the Sacred Knowledge of Life, Health, and Longevity. So many people are tired of going to the same doctor feeding them the same pills that keep them in the same cycle of illness medication repeat, it's sickening! It's almost as if we've been programmed to view our health this way when there are far better ways to do it.

Our culture has allowed the health care industry to become so powerful and disproportionately lucrative that it is now in the business of illness rather than health. So many people are tired of going to the same doctor feeding them the same pills that keep them in the same cycle of illness medication repeat, it's sickening! It's almost as if we've been programmed to view our health this way when there are far better ways to do it.

Have you ever wondered why every time you take your medication or visit the doctor's office, your illnesses seem to be getting worse? Have you ever noticed that every time you STOPPED going to the doctor for a long period of time and were off the medications, your illness, although still there, does not get any worse? That's because these medications were specifically designed by private companies and doctors alike, whose common end goal is to profit off of your illness. Wouldn't it be much wiser not to put our entire faith and trust into these people?

Most medical schools don't teach disease prevention, proper diet or exercise as a part of health. Objective measures are emphasized - white blood cell counts, blood pressure readings, etc., instead of how the patient feels. Pain is treated as a powerful enemy, its symptoms assaulted with prescription drugs that mask it or drive it underground- a practice that usually means it will resurface later with increased intensity.

The twenty-first century finds many people using more natural, less drug-oriented therapies, sometimes as an alternative to conventional medicine, sometimes in a team approach along with it. As orthodox medicine becomes more invasive, and less in touch with the person who is ill, informed people are becoming more willing to take a measure of responsibility for their own health.

Health is a lifestyle process. It is based in wellness care, instead of just illness treatment. The best news is that natural remedies work - often better than prescription drugs for many health conditions.

There are other approaches to complementary health that focus on a system, rather than just a single practice or remedy, such as massage. These systems center on a philosophy, such as the power of nature or the presence of energy in your body. Examples of these approaches include:

• Ancient healing systems. These healing systems arose long before conventional Western medicine and include Ayurveda from India and traditional Chinese medicine.

• Homeopathy. This approach uses very small doses of a drug that cause symptoms to stimulate the body's self-healing response.

• Naturopathy. This approach focuses on noninvasive treatments to help your body do its own healing and uses a variety of practices, such as massage, acupuncture, herbal remedies, exercise and lifestyle counseling.

The practices in alternative medicine make use of substances found in nature, like herbs, food, and vitamins, while modern medicine using synthetic opioids.

There is a reason a vast majority of people all over the world are beginning to shun Western medicine and are looking elsewhere, practicing alternative medicine and ingesting natural herbs due to the high epidemic of opioids going on especially in the United States of America. People all over the world are finding newer, healthier alternatives than the typical injection of pharmaceuticals which have often times been proven to do more harm than good in many cases throughout history. Follow me, and see why Billions of people worldwide are making the switch to clean, natural, organic herbs, as opposed to the usual synthetic material doctors have been force feeding us for years. This is the Revolution of the Heart, Mind, Body, Soul, and Spirit! This is the first installment in Dr. Calvin Clide's Series, Ultimate Superfoods, and in it contains the foundations of health, longevity, and nourishment. But don't take my word for it, read it yourself!

2 AMLA EXTRACT (INDIAN GOOSEBERRY)

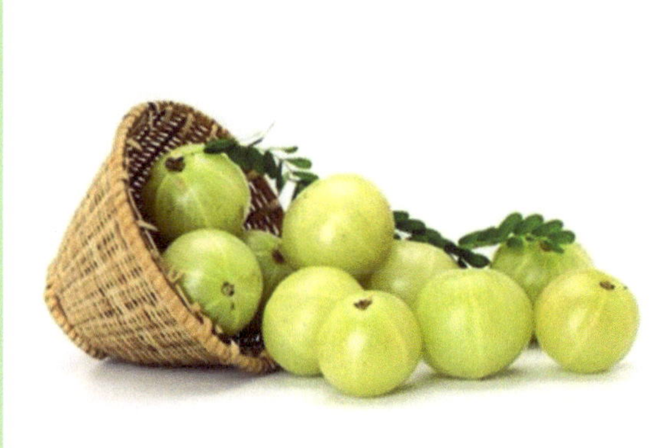

AMALAKI

VARIETY: Emblica Officinalis

Origin: India

Amla is a tart herb perfect for teas that contains the highest amount of Vitamin C of any other Ayurvedic extract in natural form.

Amla has been a very important herb in Ayurveda for more than 3,000 years. The Amla berry, also known as the Indian Gooseberry, is found on small trees that grow throughout India. The Indian Gooseberry grows on the Phyllanthus Emblica, syn. Emblica Officinalis, a deciduous tree of the Euphorbiaceae variety and it contains the highest amount of Vitamin C of any other Ayurvedic herb in natural form. Referred to in historic Ayurvedic texts as an herb promoting longevity and nourishment. You need to source a highly concentrated extract of Amla for Ayurvedic practice.

- ❖ Easy to use concentrated extract for teas and recipes.
- ❖ Referred to in historic texts as an herb promoting longevity and nourishment.
- ❖ Used in Ayurveda to enhance immunity & detoxify the body.

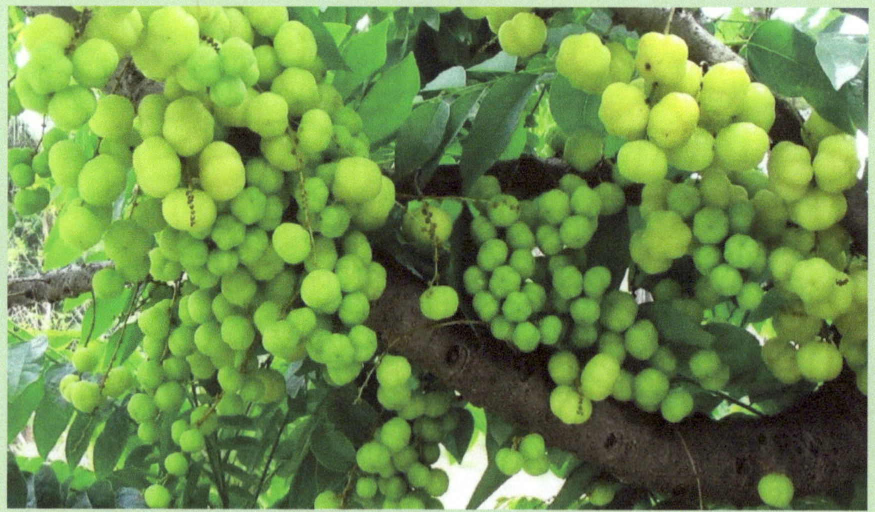

Amla is native to India, where it grows in subtropical climates, with hot, humid summers and mild winters. The tree and its fruit has been looked after by the communities in these areas for generations. The ideal growing conditions combined with years of experience result in a product high in antioxidants and is easy to incorporate into food and drink.

Process

Amla is grown throughout India in subtropical climates where the summers are hot and humid and the winters are mild. The plants are small and can take up to 6 years to bear fruit and grow up to 8 meters in height. During the fall season, the trees produce flowers that develop into smooth, round, green and yellow fruits with hard vertical stripes. The raw fruit is sour and bitter in flavor, fibrous in texture and usually mixed with other ingredients to make it more palatable.

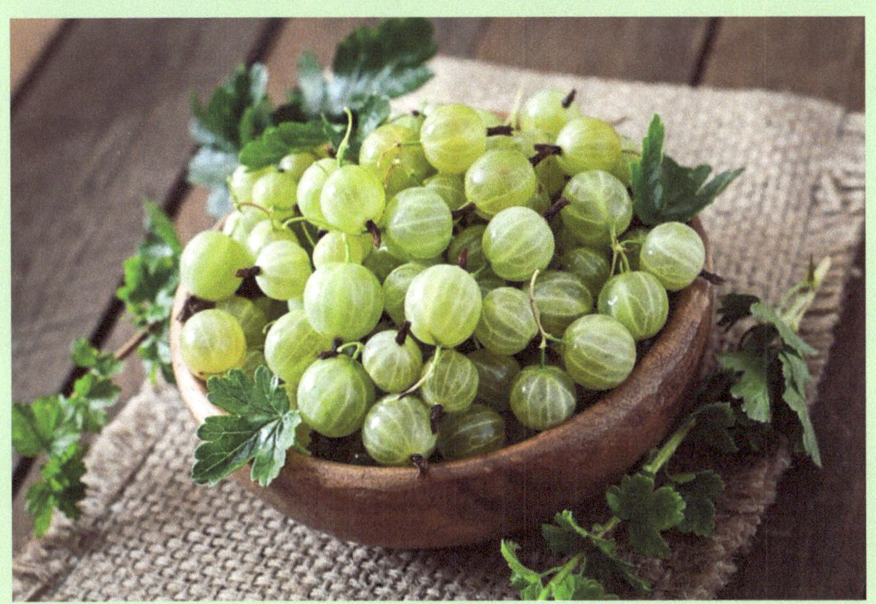

After the fruit has ripened, the berries are harvested from the upper branches of the tree and sent to be cleaned. When the amla berries are clean they are dried, ground and extracted 5:1 using pure water and ethanol. The solution is then chilled and filtered numerous times, resulting in a more concentrated product. After the amla is concentrated, it's tested and checked for quality, dried, milled and sifted.

Use

Referred to in historic Ayurvedic texts as an herb promoting longevity and nourishment.

Amla is used in Ayurveda to enhance immunity and detoxify the body. It is easy to use in concentrated extracts for teas and recipes.

Amla enhances food absorption of the body and balances stomach acid making it easier for your body to digest proteins and other fruits. It also strengthens the liver, nourishes the brain and enhances skin health.

3 BENEFITS OF AMALAKI

BENEFITS OF AMALAKI
- Supports healthy metabolism, digestion and elimination
- Promotes anti-inflammatory properties that cool, tone, and nourish tissues and organs
- Nourishes the heart and respiratory system
- Assists natural internal cleansing and maintains regularity
- Natural antioxidant
- Promotes healthy eyes, hair, nails, and skin
- Balances *agni* (digestive fire)
- Builds *ojas* to support a healthy immune response and youthfulness

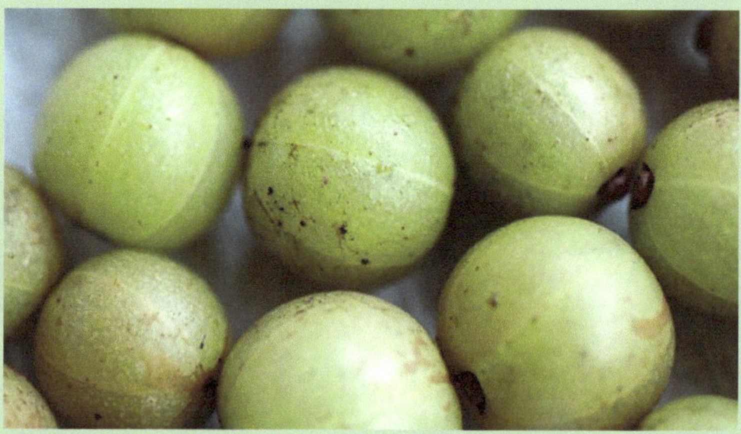

Amla literally means **"sour";** it is the Hindi word for a fruit tree (Emblica officinalis or Phyllanthus emblica) that grows throughout India and bears sour-tasting gooseberry-like fruits. Amla is also known by the Sanskrit name ***"Amalaki."*** Other Sanskrit nicknames for amla—names meaning ***"mother,"*** ***"nurse,"*** and ***"immortality"***—are a <u>testament</u> to the **healing capacity** of its fruits.

Amla has been used in Ayurveda and other Asian medicinal practices for thousands of years. Because Sanskrit is the first language of Ayurveda, it is best to refer to the herb according to its Sanskrit name and therefore offers Amla is also known as **Amalaki.**

Amla is one of the three fruits that are contained in Triphala and it is the main ingredient in the nutritive jam ***Chyavanprash***.

Amla is commonly known to contain vitamin C. Some sources even suggest that this fruit has one of the highest known concentrations of vitamin C in the plant kingdom—twenty times that of an orange.

More importantly, the vitamin C naturally found within the amla fruit is stabilized by the presence of tannins, which help amla to maintain its vitamin content even through processing.

Amla pacifies vata, pitta, and kapha, though it is especially calming to pitta.

Amla rejuvenates all of the tissues in the body and builds **_ojas;_** **_the positive subtle essence of kapha, which gives the body strength, vigor, vitality, and immunity; the end product of perfect digestion; the essence of immunity and youthfulness._** In general, Amla is a powerful ally for many systems of the body. It is known to **_promote energy, reproductive health, and healthy cholesterol levels._** Amla is **_also a tonic for the heart, the arterial system, the respiratory system, the sense organs, and the mind._**

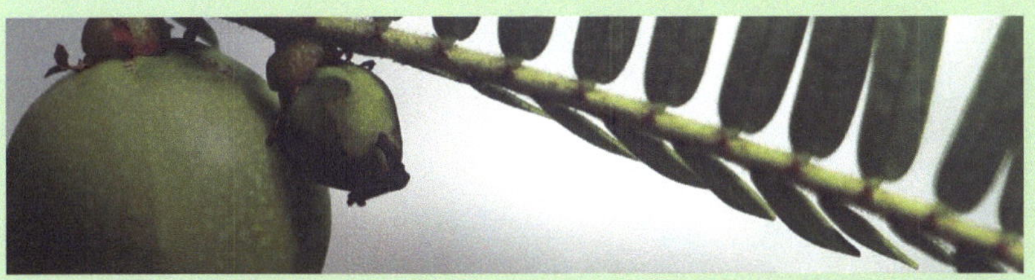

7 MAJOR BENEFITS

1) REDUCES SKIN-AGING
> ➢ Amla is considered a super fruit that is full of antioxidants which can be effective in reducing cell damage. It reduces the effects of free radicals, which are responsible for damaging protein and cell membranes.

2) FIGHTS AGAINST HEART DISEASES
> ➢ Amla reduces the buildup of bad cholesterol, which is one of the major causes of heart disease.

- ➢ Amla also reduces the risk of heart disease
- ➢ Amla reduces clogging in the arteries by boosting good cholesterol or HDL
- ➢ There are other studies which have also shown it to be effective in preventing the thickening of blood vessel walls

3) INCREASES DIURETIC ACTIVITY

- ➢ Indian gooseberry is believed to have the ability to increase the absorption of protein, a great way to boost your metabolic rate. For those of you who are unfamiliar with the term, your metabolic rate is an indicator of how fast your body burns calories. Boosting it can definitely lead to faster weight loss and stimulate higher energy levels.

4) HIGH IN DIGESTIVE FIBER

- ➢ Amla is high in fiber, water content, and has anti-inflammatory properties
- ➢ Fiber is essential for healthy bowel movements
- ➢ It is also necessary for the secretion of gastric and digestive juices
- ➢ Great for the entire digestive process

5) BOOSTS IMMUNITY

- ➢ Amla is a rich source of antioxidants, vitamins and contains tannins
- ➢ Tannins, when combined with polyphenols, make the fruit a free radical scavenger. This means that it reduces the damage free radicals cause to the cells and improves your body's disease fighting ability

6) PREVENTS ULCERS

- ➤ Amla has antibacterial properties, which makes it a great way of preventing ulcers
- ➤ This reduces the acidity level in the body, which can cause ulcers
- ➤ For example: mouth ulcers can be caused by a deficiency of Vitamin C

- ➤ As Indian gooseberries are rich in Vitamin C, they can provide relief from ulcers

7) HAIR CARE

- ➤ Amla is used in many hair tonics because it enriches hair growth and hair pigmentation
- ➤ It strengthens the root of hair, maintains color, and improves luster
- ➤ Eating fresh gooseberry or applying its paste on hair roots improves hair growth and color
- ➤ Amla can also help retain your hair's natural color and prevent it from graying

Detoxification and Healthy Elimination

Amla very directly promotes detoxification with its rich antioxidant content.

On a systemic level, detoxification begins with healthy *Agni (digestive fire)*, not only in the GI tract, but also in all of the tissues, and Amla helps to balance Agni throughout the body. Moreover, the elimination of toxins relies on *healthy circulation, digestion, and elimination,* and Amla supports all three of these functions.

Amla also has a particular affinity for the blood, the liver, and the spleen, and is therefore able to *support the elimination of natural toxins while nourishing and protecting the body's natural defense systems.*

Proper elimination is critically important to the detoxification process and *Amla fosters bowel health and regularity as well.*

A small dose of Amla is binding and astringent in its effect while a larger dose very gently encourages elimination.

Ultimately, Amla supports virtually every stage of the detoxification process—from the innate intelligence of Agni to the proper elimination of wastes and natural toxins.

Digestion

From an Ayurvedic perspective, digestion begins with the experience of taste and *Amla contains five of the six tastes, lacking only the salty taste.* Further, Amla *sharpens the sense of taste itself* and so it is *both stimulating and tonifying to the first stage of digestion.* Amla also *improves appetite and kindles Agni (the digestive fire), which are both at the core of healthy digestion.*

Despite the fact that its predominant taste is sour, *Amla stokes the digestive fire without aggravating pitta.* And, *Amla cleanses and protects the liver, which plays a critical role in transforming food into physiologically useful nourishment.* Because pitta and Agni are so intimately connected, the health of the digestive fire suffers when pitta is aggravated.

Amla is particularly suited to clearing excess pitta from the digestive tract; its bitter taste and cooling energy help to flush excess heat out through the bowel.

Amla can be especially supportive to digestion during the summer months when heat tends to accumulate in the body, particularly for those with pitta-predominant constitutions.

Healthy Blood Sugar Levels

Amla's ability to ***stimulate microcirculation*** and to build ojas are ***thought to help promote healthy blood sugar levels, particularly in conjunction with pitta imbalances.***

Amla also has an affinity for the urinary tract and balanced excretion of urine and balanced blood sugar levels go hand in hand. On a large scale***, Amla's support of the entire digestive process supports the body's ability to process food in a wholesome and efficient manner.***

Rejuvenation

Amla is a highly revered rasayana ***(rejuvenative) for the entire system.*** Specifically***, it promotes youthfulness, bolsters immunity, tonifies all the body's tissues and promotes overall health and well-being.***

It is a brain tonic, it promotes memory, and its sattvic nature fosters subtle awareness, balanced emotions, and clarity of mind.

4 TRIPHALA

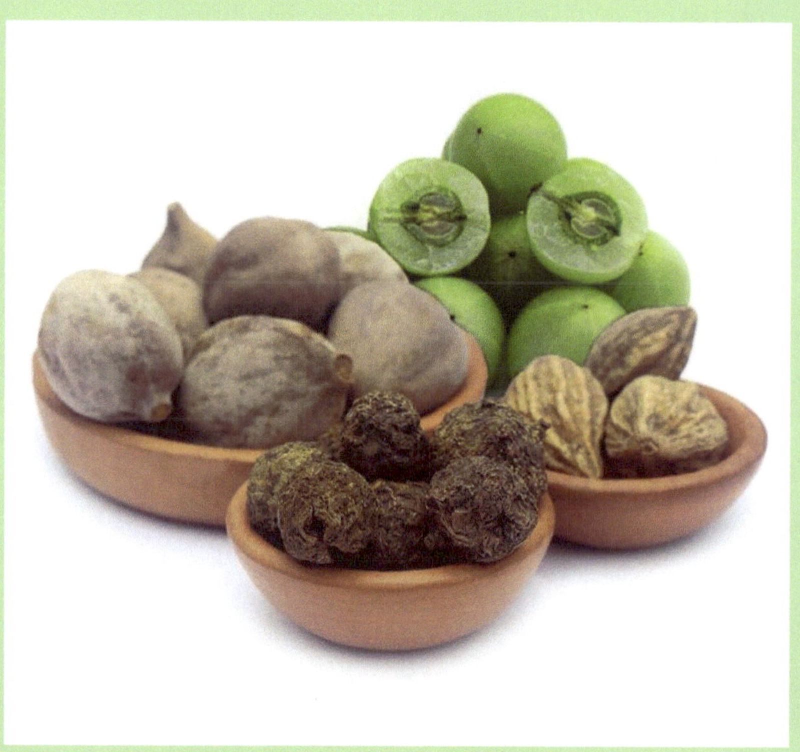

Triphala literally means *'three fruits'* and includes equal portions (by weight) of **Amla, Bibhitaki, and Haritaki.**

Triphala is the most widely used formula in Ayurveda. Like Amla, *Triphala contains five of the six tastes—all but salty—and is primarily used to maintain a healthy digestive tract.*

Triphala is deeply nourishing and cleansing to all tissues and is a very effective detoxifier.

Triphala also benefits the lungs, skin, and eyes, and it can be used as part of a weight loss program that includes proper diet and exercise.

Triphala is typically taken as a hot infusion at night or as a cold infusion upon rising. *If there are clear signs of excess heat and inflammation in the digestive tract, Amla taken alone may prove more supportive than Triphala.*

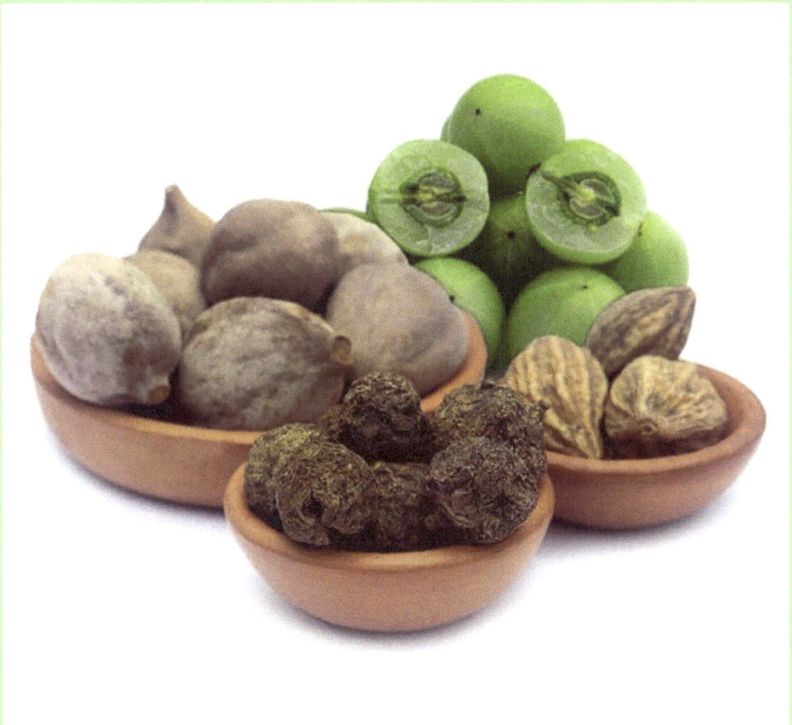

5 CHYAVANPRASH

Amla in Chyavanprash

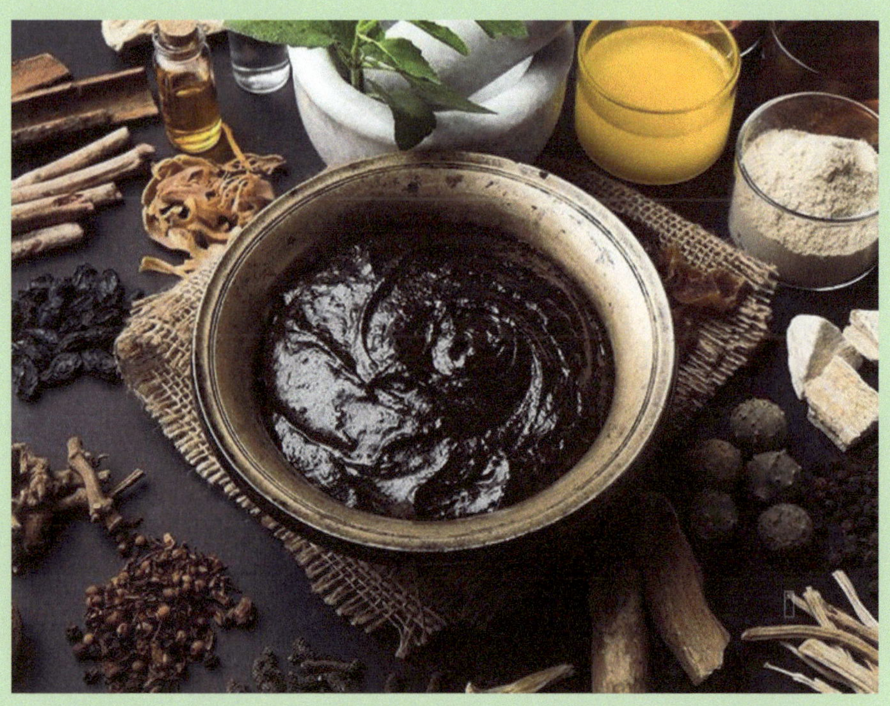

Chyavanprash is a delicious nutritive jam, primarily

aimed at bolstering the immune system. Chyavanprash is made with a base of fresh Amla fruits and also includes a number of other herbs, ghee, sesame oil, sugar, and/or honey. It is particularly *supportive of the respiratory tract as it nourishes the mucous membranes and helps keep the respiratory passages clean and clear.*

Chyavanprash also strengthens vata, nourishes the reproductive tissues, aides in the elimination of ama (toxins), and builds ojas.

Chyavanprash can be taken on a long-term basis as part of a program designed to support overall strengthening, or recovery from an illness or stress.

For others, it is more appropriately used seasonally, as a **tonic** in the winter months.

Taking Chyavanprash in milk (or almond milk if dairy is not appropriate) helps to carry its tonifying and rejuvenating qualities deep into the tissues.

6 SOURCE

Located south east of China, India is an extremely large country with diverse climates and terrains. The Tropic of Cancer passes through the middle of India, making most of India's climate topical with unpredictable weather. The landscape ranges from miles of coastline to the Himalayan Mountains which separate the northern part of the country from China.

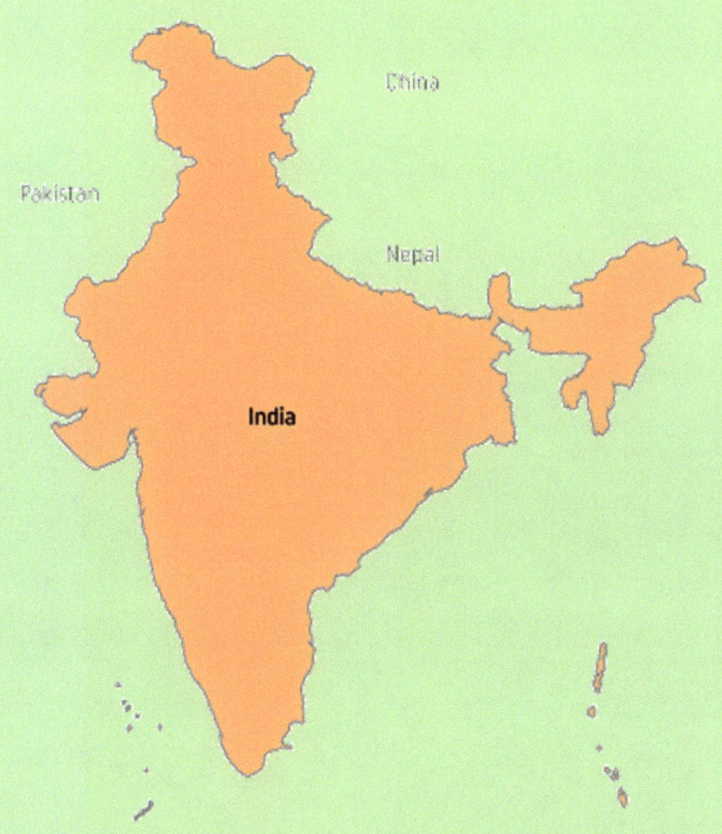
China
Pakistan
Nepal
India

7 THE AMLA TREE

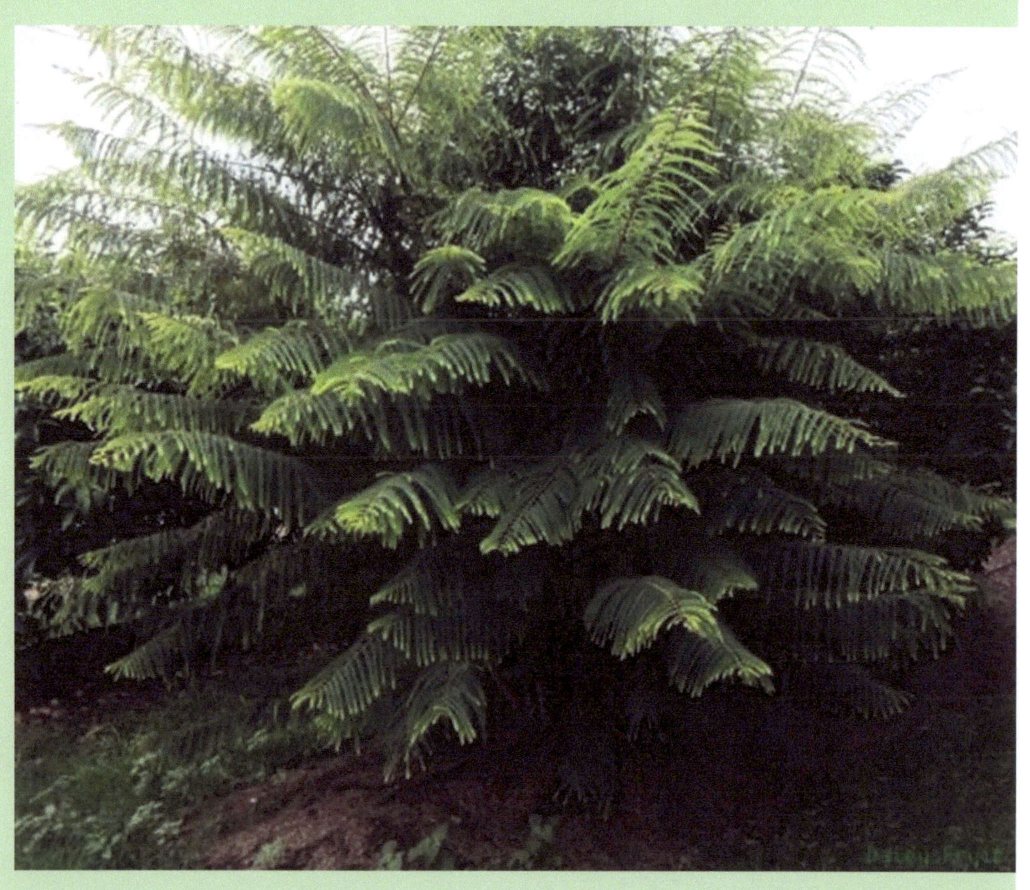

Phyllanthus Emblica, also known as emblic, emblic myrobalan, myrobalan, Indian gooseberry, Malacca tree, or Amla from Sanskrit Amalaki - a deciduous tree of the family Phyllanthaceae. It has edible fruit, referred to by the same name.

The tree is considered sacred by Hindus as a deity, Vishnu, is believed to dwell in it. The tree is worshipped on Amalaka Ekadashi.

In other Hindu beliefs, Amla is said to have originated from the drops of Amrit which spilled on earth accidentally, because of the fight of gods and demons after ksheera sagar manthan. This religious belief makes claims that it almost cures every disease and is also good in extending the longevity of life.
In the Sanskrit Buddhist tradition, half an amalaka fruit was the final gift to the Buddhist sangha by the great Indian emperor Ashoka. This is illustrated in the Ashokavadana in the following verses:
"A great donor, the lord of men, the eminent Maurya Ashoka, has gone from being lord of Jambudvipa [the continent] to being lord of half a myrobalan" (Strong, 1983, p. 99). This deed became so famous that a stupa was created to mark the place of the event in modern-day Patna and was known as the Amalaka stupa.

According to Hindu tradition, Adi Shankara of Kerala composed and recited the Kanakadhara stotram in praise of Mahalakshmi to help a poor Brahmin lady obtain wealth, in return for a single amla presented to him as bhiksha on an auspicious Dwadashi day.

According to a Tamil legend, Avvaiyar, a female poet, ethicist and political activist of the Sangam period was gifted with one nellikkai by King Athiyaman to give her long life.

Amalaka at the top of the Lingaraj temple in Bhubaneswar

In Theravada Buddhism, this plant is said to have been used as the tree for achieving enlightenment, or Bodhi by twenty first Buddha named Phussa Buddha.

In Indian temple architecture, an amalaka is a stone disk, usually with ridges on the rim, that sits atop a temple's main tower (Shikhara). The shape of the amalaka is thought to have been inspired by the fruit of the Amla tree.

In traditional Indian medicine, dried and fresh fruits of the plant are used. All parts of the plant are used in various Ayurvedic medicine herbal preparations, including the fruit, seed, leaves, root, bark and flowers. According to Ayurveda, Amla fruit is sour (amla) and astringent (Kashaya) in taste (rasa), with sweet (Madhura), bitter (Tikta) and pungent (Katu) secondary tastes (Anurasas). Its qualities (Gunas) are light (Laghu) and dry (Ruksha), the postdigestive effect (Vipaka) is sweet (Madhura) and its energy (Virya) is cooling (Shita).

In Ayurvedic polyherbal formulations, Indian gooseberry is a common constituent, and most notably is the primary ingredient in an ancient herbal rasayana called Chyavanprash.

Pratapgarh is one of the largest producers and suppliers of Indian gooseberries. In this region, the fruit is commonly pickled with salt, oil, and spices. The amla fruit is eaten raw or cooked into various dishes. In Pratapgarh, tender varieties are used to prepare dal (a lentil preparation), and amle ka murabbah, a sweet dish made by soaking the berries in sugar syrup until they are candied. It is traditionally consumed after meals.
In the Batak area of Sumatra, Indonesia, the inner bark is used to impart an astringent, bitter taste to the broth of a traditional fish soup known as holat.

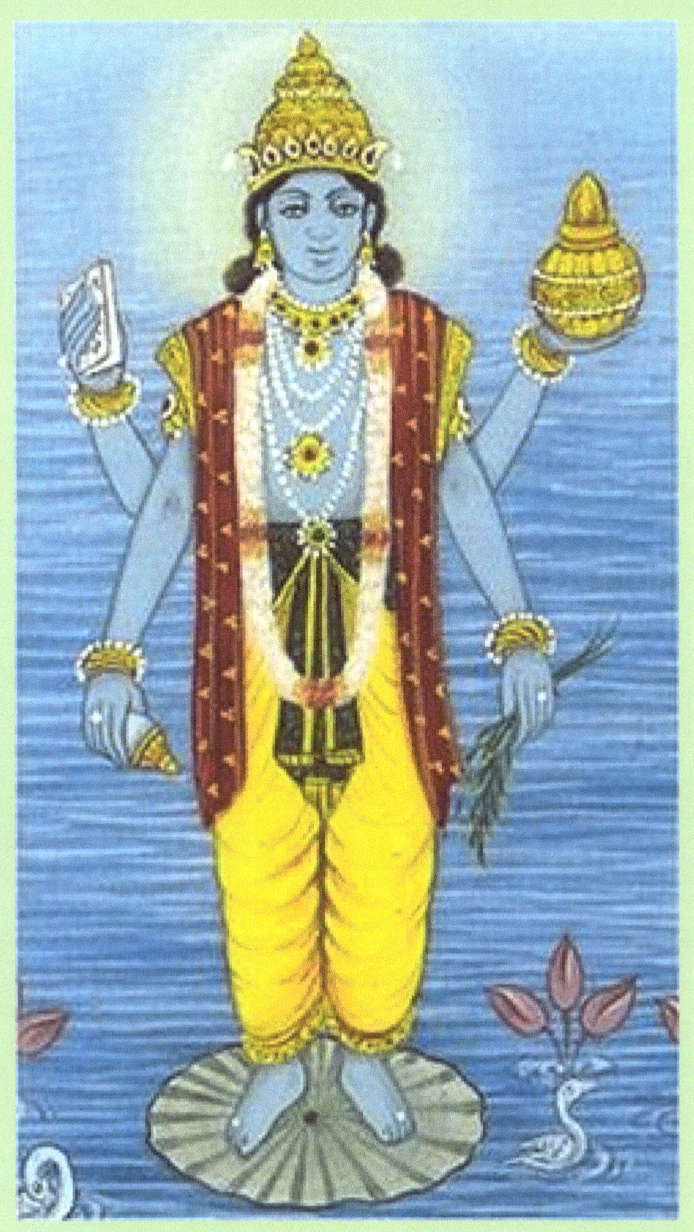

Dhanwantari
God of Ayurveda
Physician of the Gods
and Doctors

A small to medium sized deciduous tree, 8-18m. in height with crooked trunk and spreading branches. Leaves simple, sub sessile; flower greenish-yellow; fruit nearly spherical pale yellow with 6 vertical furrows.

COMMON NAMES: Amlaki, Indian gooseberry, Anola, Amlika.

DISTRIBUTION :

A moderate-sized deciduous tree found wild or planted throughout the deciduous forests of tropical India and on hill slopes up to 2000m.

PART USED: Fruit.

CULTIVATION:

SOIL AND CLIMATE

Amla can be grown in light as well as heavy soils except purely sandy soil. Calcareous soil with rocky substratum can also be good. However, well drained fertile loamy soil is the best for higher yield. The plant have capacity for adaptation to dry regions and can also grow in moderately alkaline soils.

It is grown extensively under tropical condition. Annual rainfall of 630-800 mm have given good yield. The young plants up to the age of 3 years should be protected from hot wind during May-June and from frost during winter months. The mature plants can tolerate freezing temperature as well as temperature up to 46^0C.

Nursery Raising and Planting

Amla is generally propagated through seeds, but seed propagated trees bear inferior quality fruits and have a long gestation period. Shield budding is done on one year old seedlings with buds collected from superior strains yielding big size fruits. Older trees of inferior types can be rejuvenated and easily changed into superior type by top working.

The pits of $1m^3$ are prepared during May-June at a distance of 4.5 m spacing and should be left for 15-20 days exposed to sunlight. Each pit should be filled with surface soil mixed with 15 kg farm yard manure and one kg of super phosphate before planting the grafted seedling.

WEEDING AND HOEING

Weeding & Hoeing is required in nursery.

MANURES, FERTILISERS AND PESTICIDES

The medicinal plants have to be grown without chemical fertilizers and use of pesticides. Organic manures like, Farm Yard Manure (FYM), Vermi-Compost, Green Manure etc. may be used as per requirement of the species. To prevent diseases, bio-pesticides could be prepared (either single or mixture) from Neem (kernel, seeds & leaves), Chitrakmool, Dhatura, Cow's urine etc.

IRRIGATION

https://www.nmpb.nic.in/sites/default/files/publications/amla.pdf

27

Amla plants hardly require irrigation during monsoon. Young plants require watering during summer months at 15 days interval till they have fully established. Watering of mature fruit bearing plants is advised during summer months at bi-weekly intervals to increase fruit set and to reduce fruit drop. It responds very well to drip irrigation. After the monsoon rains, during October-December about 25-30 litres of water per day per tree through drips should be given.

HARVESTING/POST HARVESTING OPERATION

Amla seedlings start bearing fruits in 7-8 years after planting, while the budded clones will start bearing fruits from the 5th year onwards. The fruits are light green at first, but when they mature become dull greenish yellow. Best harvesting time of Amla fruits is February when the fruits have maximum ascorbic acid content. In South India, fruits are found throughout the year. The mature fruits are hard and they do not fall for gentle touch and therefore vigorous shaking is required. For getting attractive prices fruits after harvest should be made into different grades depending on the size. Fruits can also be harvested using long bamboo poles attached with hooks.

YIELD

A matured tree of about 10 years will yield 50-70 kg of fruit. The average weight of the fruits is 60-70 g. One kg contains about 1`5-20 number of fruits. A well maintained tree will be yielding up to an age of 70 years. The yield increases year by year up to 50 years.

ECONOMICS

The 8-year old plantation of one hectare will yield 20-25 tons of fruits with a cost of production of Rs.34,000 per-ha. The rate for a kg of fruit Rs.15-30.

Net income- per hectare: Rs.20,000/-(YEAR-2001)

NOTE: MARKET FOR MEDICINAL PLANTS IS VOLATILE AND THE ECONOMICS MAY VARY.

8 HOW TO USE AMLA

Because taste plays such an important role in the digestive process and signals the body to initiate its own supportive mechanisms, Ayurveda traditionally recommends tasting herbs. Amla can be taken internally in four forms: *a powder, a tablet, a liquid extract, or in a jam such as Chyavanprash.*

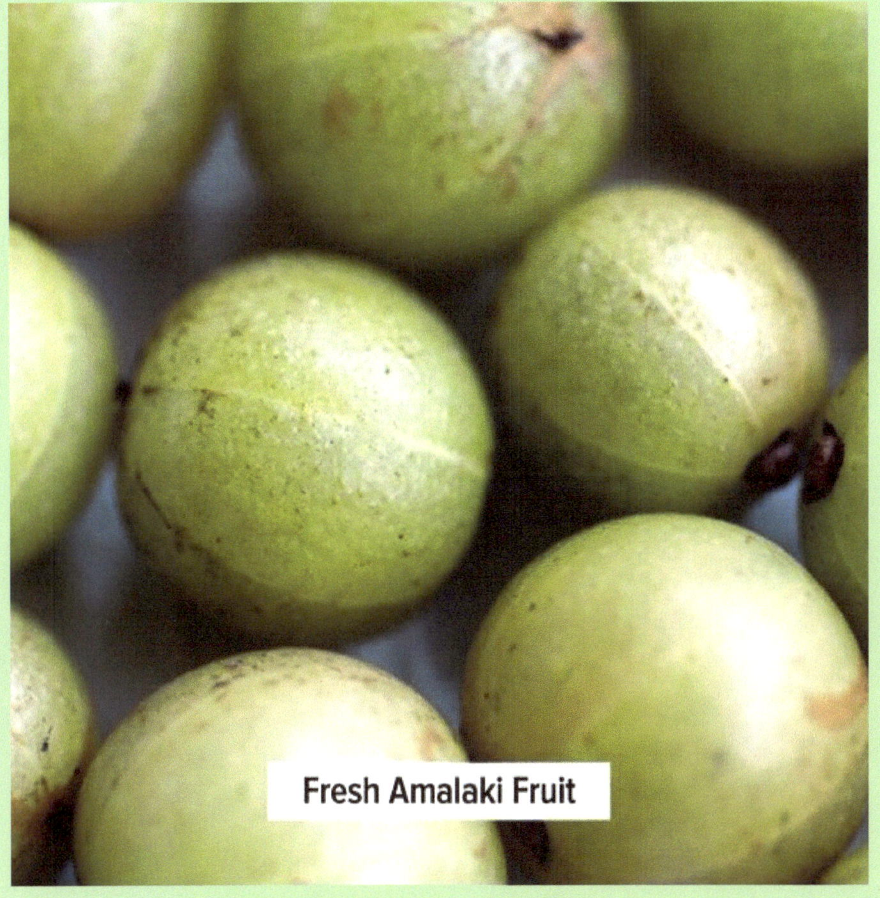

Fresh Amalaki Fruit

9 AMLA POWDER

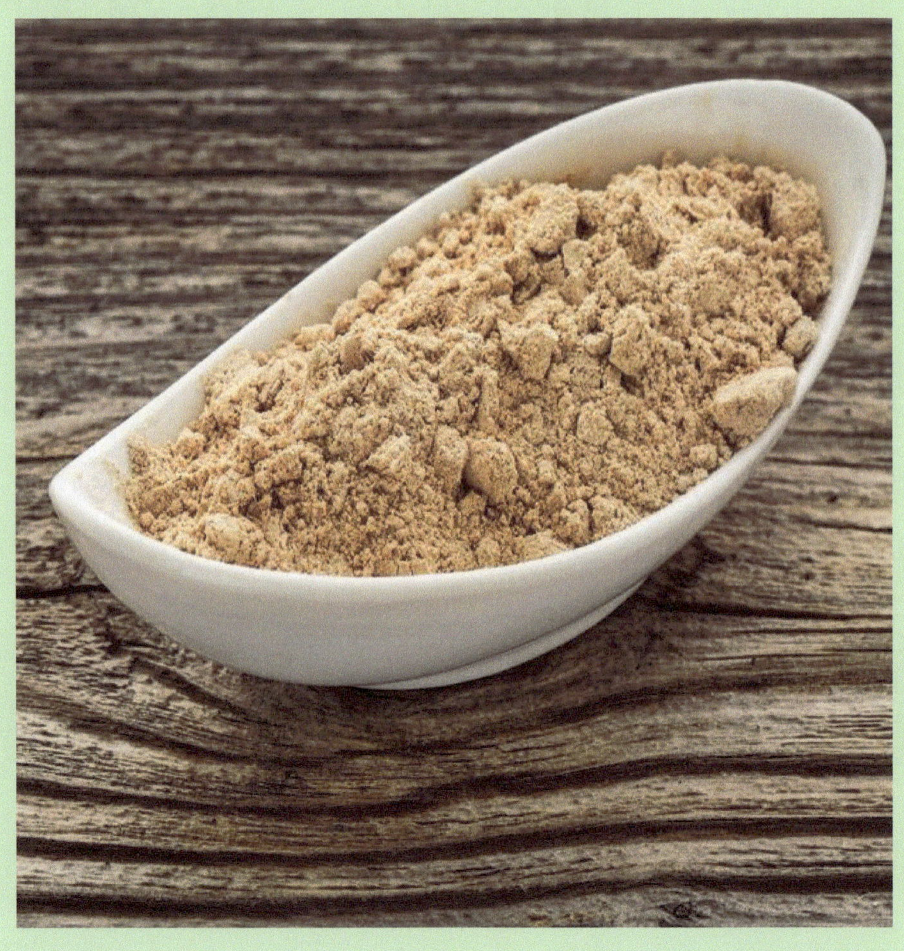

Amla powder offers the full experience of tasting the herb and also provides the most economical option for purchasing Amla.

Like Triphala, Amla powder can be taken as a hot or cold infusion in water, at night or upon rising.

In some instances, taking Amla in milk, ghee or another carrier substance may help to direct the herb to a specific tissue or organ, or guide it toward a particular kind of systemic support.

An Ayurvedic practitioner can advise you on the appropriate ***Anupan (carrier)*** for your herbs.

You can also refer to the Ayurveda's Carrier Substances guide to better understand which Anupan is most appropriate for you.

A typical dose of Amla powder is ¼–½ teaspoon, once or twice daily, or as directed by your healthcare practitioner.

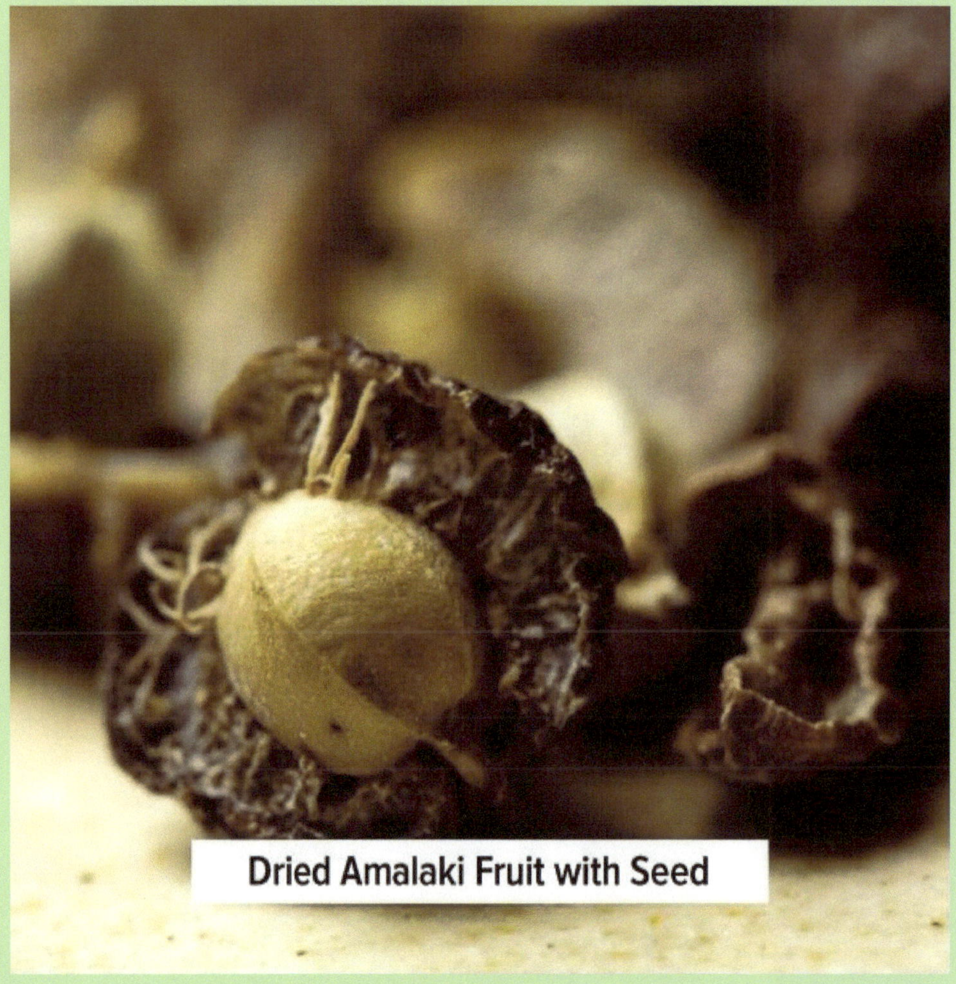

Dried Amalaki Fruit with Seed

10 AMLA TABLETS

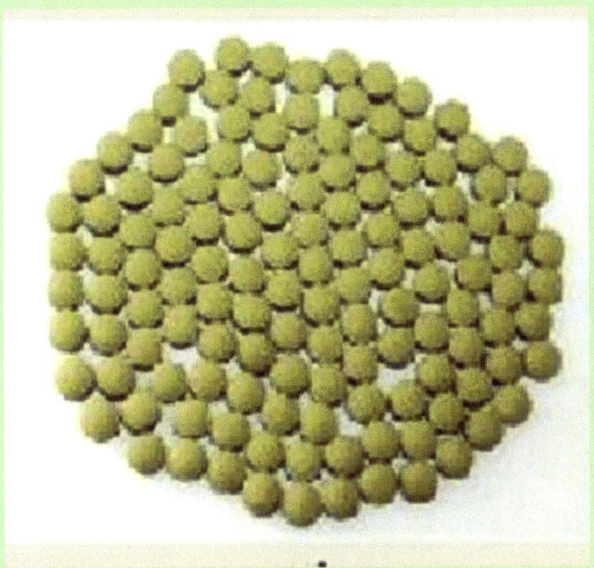

100% USDA Organic tablets provide a more convenient way to take Amla, especially for those who are frequently traveling or on the go.

The tablets also provide a nice alternative for those who find the taste a deterrent to taking the herb.

It is provided in a tablet form (rather than a capsule) because tablets allow you to get a sample of the taste, allowing the digestive process to receive appropriate signals about what you are about to ingest and inviting the body to initiate other healing mechanisms.

A typical dose is one to two tablets, once or twice daily, or as directed by your healthcare practitioner.

11 AMLA LIQUID EXTRACT

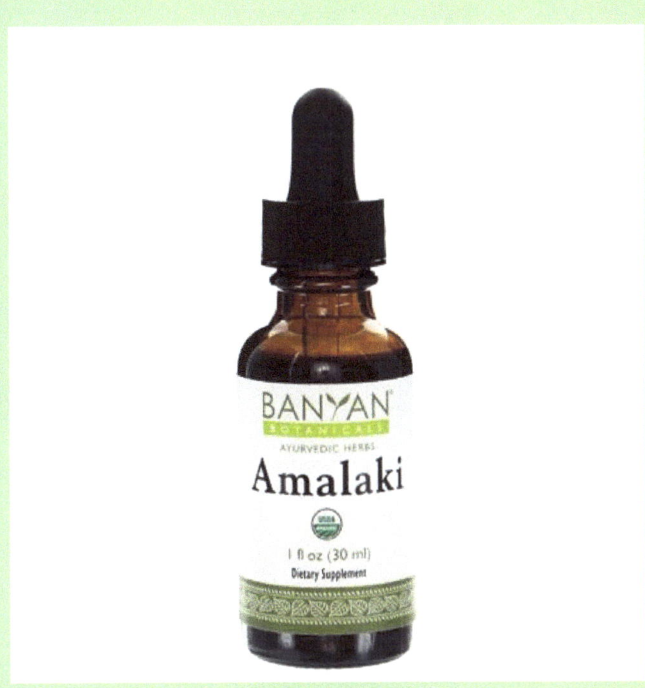

Amla liquid extract provides an alternative method of taking Amla. ***It's convenient, easy to assimilate, and has a long shelf life.*** This extract is made from the same certified organic Amla used in making the herbal tablets and is extracted using non-GMO, gluten-free grain alcohol.

A typical dose is a dropper full (about 30 drops) taken in 1–2 ounces of water or juice, one to three times daily, or as directed by your healthcare practitioner.

12 AMLA IN A NUTRITIVE JAM - CHYVANPRASH

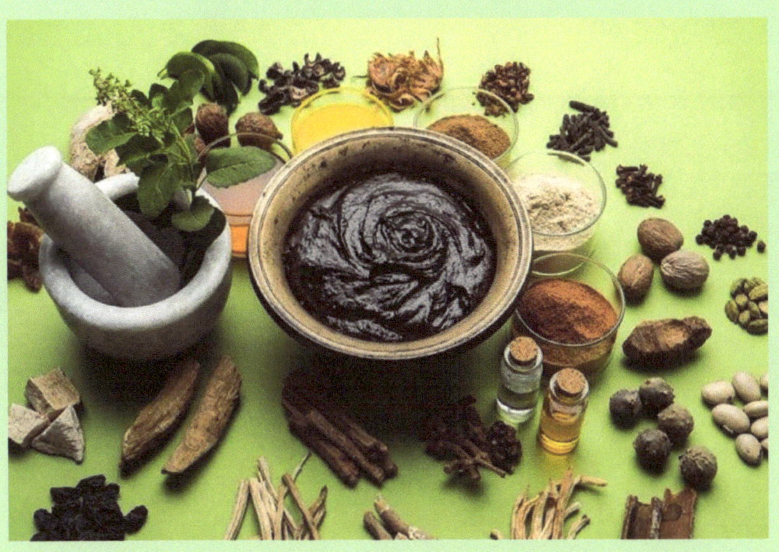

As a *rejuvenative*, Chyavanprash is *typically taken in the morning and evening.*

Chyavanprash is a tasty jam, and as such *offers the full experience of tasting the herbal ingredients.*

The usual dose of chyavanprash is 1–3 teaspoons, once or twice daily, or as directed by your healthcare practitioner.

13 MODERN RESEARCH ON AMLA

There has been significant scientific research evaluating the benefits of Amla both on its own, and as an ingredient in Chyavanprash and Triphala. Among other things, *studies have looked at Amla's ability to foster appropriate glucose levels, cholesterol levels, and its immunomodulatory and antioxidant effects.* Below are a few links that summarize some of these findings:

- Effect of Chyavanprash and Vitamin C on Glucose Tolerance and Lipoprotein Profile. PubMed Abstract. Jan 2001.
- Effect of the Indian Gooseberry (Amla) on Serum Cholesterol Levels in Men Aged 35-55 Years. PubMed Abstract. Nov 1988.
- Immunomodulatory effects of agents of plant origin. PubMed Abstract. Sep 2003.

Cytotoxic Response of Breast Cancer Cell Lines, MCF 7 and T 47 D to Triphala and its Modification by Antioxidants. PubMed Abstract. Jul 2006.

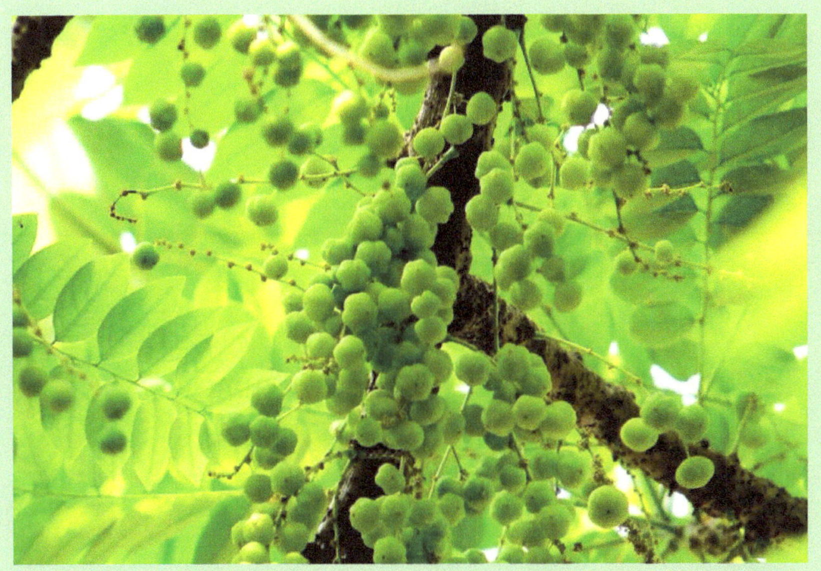

SIDE EFFECTS &
CONTRAINDICATIONS

Side Effects

A night dose of Amla before sleep can weaken the teeth in the same way that over-exposure to citrus fruits might erode tooth enamel; taken in this manner, Amla may also irritate the throat. Being an edible fruit, <u>there are no other known issues with Amla, even at higher doses.</u>

Contraindications

Amla should be avoided in cases of high **Ama (toxicity)** or when **kapha** is especially aggravated. It is also ill advised when individuals of a pitta-predominant constitution have diarrhea. *There is some evidence to suggest caution among individuals with an iron deficiency because Amla can form chelates with iron and thus reduce the amount of usable iron in the blood. Traditionally* however, Amla *has been used to balance and build the blood.*

DISCLAIMER

When purchasing Amla and products containing Amla, there are a number of questions to consider that will help you to evaluate the quality of the herbs, the values upheld by the company that produced them, and the price of the product in relation to its quality.

Is the supplier able to trace the ingredients of their product back to the fields in which they were grown?

Traceability of the herbs from field to shelf allows the supplier to know where and how the herbs were grown and when they were harvested. It is best to know exactly where each ingredient was grown and trace them back from your medicine cabinet to the field.

Is the Amla grown in optimal locations?

Location does play a role in quality. Like the grapes in wine, herbs tend to vary in quality and taste depending on the conditions in which they are grown. Make sure your supplier sources Amla from areas where the trees thrive naturally.

Are the ingredients sustainably harvested?

Amla is relatively abundant in many parts of India. Where and how it is harvested makes a big difference in sustainability. Amla can be harvested on private farms where sustainability can be managed, or it may be wild-harvested from the forest legally. Sometimes, it is wild-harvested illegally, threatening long-term sustainability. Ensure sustainability by sourcing the Amla used in its products from privately owned farms where it has been cultivated. The fruits are harvested at optimal times, using environmentally sustainable practices that are sensitive to the long-term health of the trees and their surrounding ecosystems.

Are the farmers looked after for their labor?

Harvesting and processing Amla is labor intensive. Find a supplier that strongly believes in maintaining socially responsible relationships with farmers and committed to following fair trade principles which include paying above-market wages, investing in the education of the farmers, and giving back to their communities.

Are the ingredients organic?

This is an especially important consideration when choosing an herb for medicinal benefits.

When an herb contains genetic alterations or toxic residues from chemical pesticides, the very substance that was intended to support health and healing can be harmful. Buying organic herbs is the safest way to protect your body from these potentially dangerous toxins.

The Amla should be USDA certified organic. Please ensure that organic farming practices are adhered to.

Your supplier should receive the ingredients from trusted sources whose methods have been verified and monitored.

You can rest assured that Amla sourced through the right supplier will be free of pesticides and other harmful chemicals.

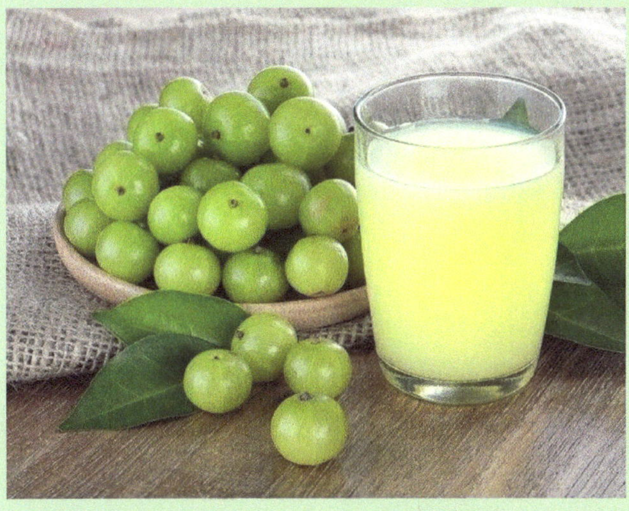

REFERENCES

1. Pole, Sebastian. *Ayurvedic Medicine: The Principles of Traditional Practice. Churchill Livingston Elsevier, 2006. 52, 126-127, 296, 303-304, 326.*

2. Gogte, Vaidya V. M. *Ayurvedic Pharmacology & Therapeutic Uses of Medicinal Plants. Reprint. Chaukhambha Publications, 2009. 310.*

3. Amalaki (Phyllanthus Emblica)." *Natural Standard: Professional Monograph. Online. 26 Feb. 2012.* http://naturalstandard.com/databases/herbssupplements/amalaki.asp

4. Manjunatha, S., et al. "Effect of Chyavanprash and Vitamin C on Glucose Tolerance and Lipoprotein Profile." *Indian Journal of Physiology and Pharmacology. 45.1 (2001): 71-79. Online. PubMed. 26 Feb. 2012.* http://www.ncbi.nlm.nih.gov/pubmed/11211574?dopt=Abstract

5. Jacob, A., et al. "Effect of the Indian Gooseberry (Amla) on Serum Cholesterol Levels in Men Aged 35-55 Years." *European Journal of Clinical Nutrition.* 42.11 (1988): 939-944. Online. PubMed. 26 Feb. 2012. http://www.ncbi.nlm.nih.gov/pubmed/3250870?dopt=Abstract

6. Ganju, L., et al. "Immunomodulatory Effects of Agents of Plant Origin." *Biomedicine & Pharmacotherapy.* 57.7 (2003): 296-300. Online. PubMed. 26 Feb. 2012. http://www.ncbi.nlm.nih.gov/pubmed/14499177?dopt=Abstract

7. Sandhya, T. and K.P. Mishra. "Cytotoxic Response of Breast Cancer Cell Lines, MCF 7 and T 47 D to Triphala and Its Modification by Antioxidants." *Cancer Letters.* 238.2 (2006): 304-313. Online. PubMed. 26 Feb. 2012. http://www.ncbi.nlm.nih.gov/pubmed/16135398?dopt=Abstract

Amla

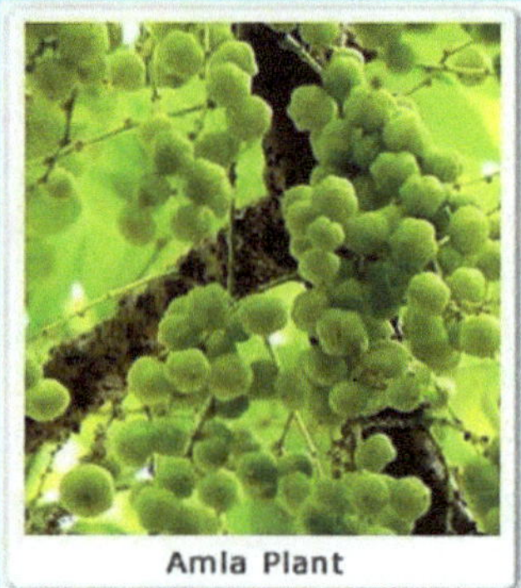

Amla Plant

- ***Other names :*** Indian gooseberry, Bhumi amla, Bhumyamalki, Amlaki, adiphala, dhatri, amalaka, amali, amalakamu, usirikai, Anola, Amlika, nellikai, malacca tree, nillika, nellikya, emblic are the other names used for the Amla.

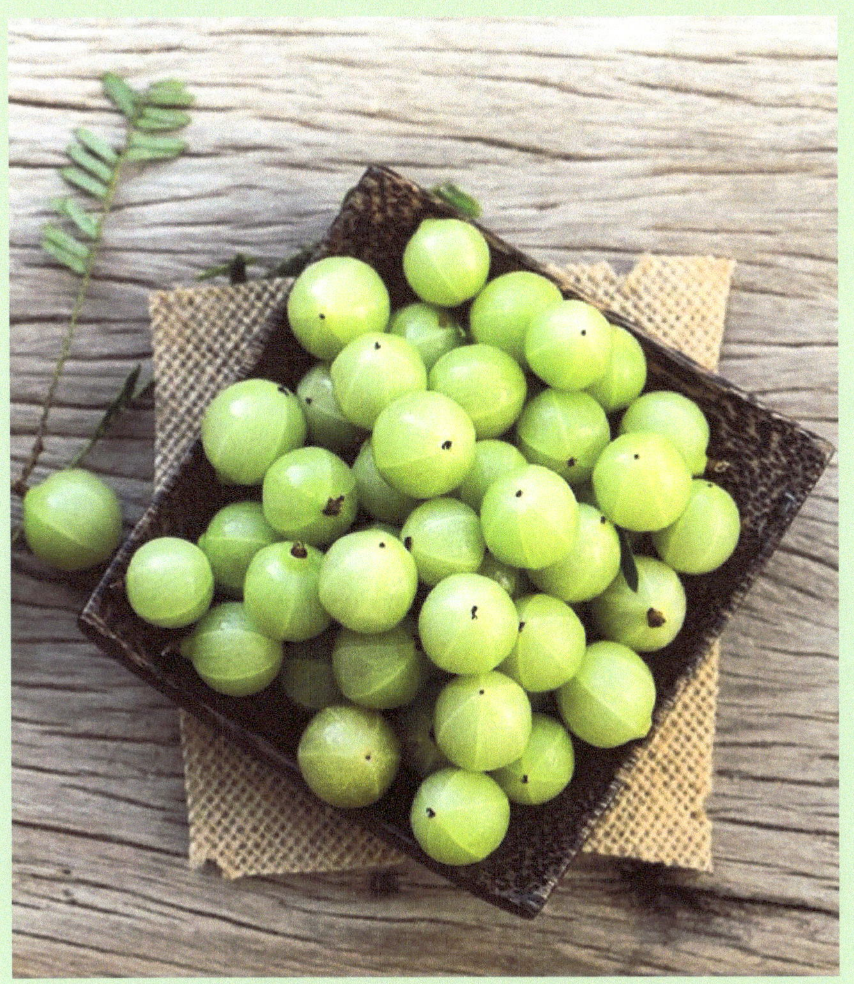

TO BE CONTINUED…

I AM DR. CALVIN CLIDE, PH.D

I have dedicated my life towards helping people heal and find new ways to better themselves whether it be self-improvement, entrepreneurship, health and fitness, dieting, nutrition, and spirituality. My main goal on this Earth is to provide knowledge and insight to those left in the dark by major corporations who seek to take advantage of their lack of knowledge and charge them and upcharge them on services and products. There is none more sinister and more detrimental to our planet than the healthcare industry, and its BIG PHARMA tycoons which have successfully fooled the entire world into buying their harmful synthetic products (opioids), and trusting their doctors when they should be taking matters into their own hands. What I teach is simple, long term health and nutrition to promote longevity and PREVENT these illnesses from happening, so that YOU do not have to visit these SICK doctors, who profit off the weak and ill-informed. This a major reason I wrote ULTIMATE SUPERFOODS, and have divided it into many volumes for the masses to easily comprehend. Follow me on my journey as I set out to heal the world, one book at a time.